Fit and Healthy

Mediterranean Cookbook

Easy and Delicious Recipes to

Improve your Health

Ben Cooper

Table of Contents

Hollandaise Sauce

Preparation Time: 10 minutes
Cooking Time: 5 minutes
Servings: 1

Ingredients:

1 lemon (Zested and juiced)
1 tsp garlic powder
1/2 tsp cayenne pepper
1/2 cup cashew butter
2 tsp Dijon mustard
1/2 cup of warm water
1/2 tsp ground turmeric

Directions:

1.In a food processor, put all ingredients, and then pulse until smooth.

2.Put it in a sealed container and refrigerate it for up to three days.

3.Enjoy.

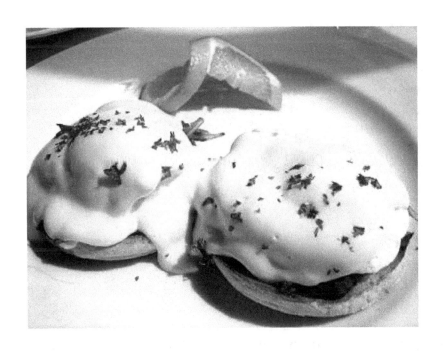

Creamy Tahini Dip

Preparation Time: 5 minutes

Cooking Time: 4 minutes

Servings: 4

Ingredients:

Half a lemon (Juiced)
1 crushed garlic clove
Salt
1/2 cup tahini
2 cups of water
Fresh parsley, chopped
Black pepper

Directions:

1.Put the tahini, salt, lemon juice, garlic, and a little water in a bowl then stir until the tahini becomes white and smooth.

2.Sprinkle the parsley and black pepper and serve.

3.Enjoy.

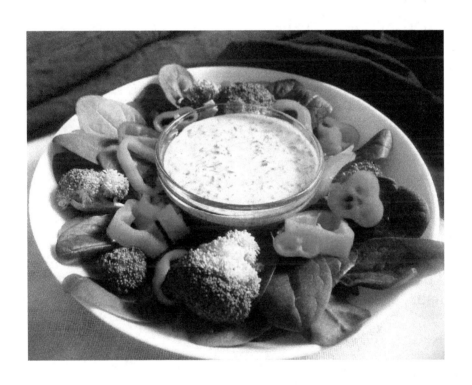

Basil Lime

Preparation Time: 5 minutes
Cooking Time: 10 minutes
Servings: 16

Ingredients:

10 garlic cloves, crushed
1/4 cup brown rice syrup
8 oz. hemp oil
1 tsp of sea salt
1 pinch xanthan gum
1 1/2 cups chopped basil,
6 tbsp key lime juice

Directions:

1.In an airtight jar, put all the ingredients except the xanthan gum, and then shake to well.

2.Put the mixture plus the xanthan, into a blender and pulse.

3.Return the mixture in the jar.

4. Enjoy.

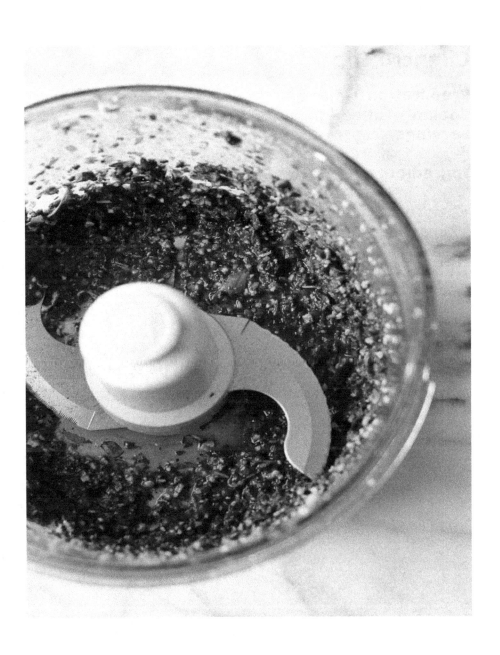

Cilantro Dip

Preparation Time: 5 minutes
Cooking Time: 4 minutes
Servings: 7

Ingredients:

12 cloves of garlic
4 cups cilantro leaves
1 tsp salt
1/2 tsp ground black pepper
1 cup olive oil

Directions:

1.Add all ingredients to a blender and pulse until velvety.

2.You can put in the refrigerator for up to two days.

3.Enjoy.

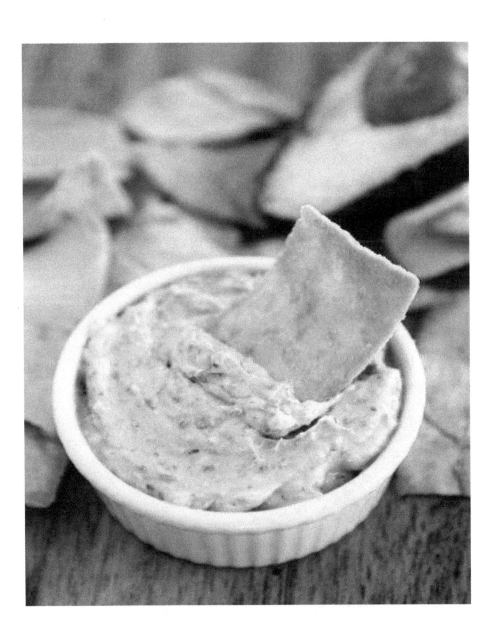

Tahini Sauce

Preparation Time: 7 minutes
Cooking Time: 5 minutes
Servings: 6

Ingredients:

4 mashed garlic cloves
Salt to taste
1 cup tahini paste
1/2 cup lemon juice
7 tbsp water

Directions:

1.Put all ingredients in a bowl and whisk until well combined.

2.Refrigerate up to 5 days.

3.Enjoy.

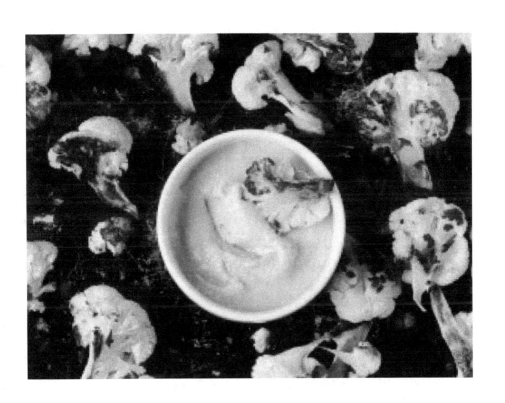

Arugula Salsa

Preparation Time: 5 minutes
Cooking Time: 20 minutes
Servings: 6

Ingredients:

30 Kalamata olives, pitted, quartered
3 tbsp olive oil
1 chopped red bell pepper
1 chopped yellow bell pepper
2 tsp fennel seeds, crushed
1 cup baby arugula, chopped

Directions:

1.Heat oil in a pan over medium heat.

2.Add fennel seeds and sauté until fragrant.

3.Add bell peppers and sauté until they are soft.

4.Transfer into a bowl.

5.Add salt, pepper, and arugula and stir until arugula wilts.

6.Enjoy.

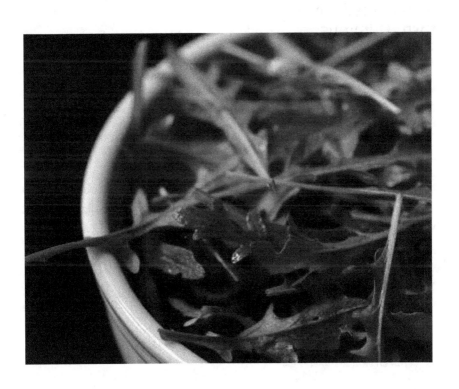

19

Mediterranean Turkey Pinwheels

Total Time: 5 minutes
Serving: 4

Ingredients:

½ cup Grated carrots
3 tbsp. Hummus
6 Pitted olives
2 Thin slices of turkey
1 Whole-Grain Flat-out Flatbread (or whole-wheat tortilla)

Directions:

1.Place the flatbread on your work surface and using a butter knife, generously spread the hummus to cover the flatbread.

2.Sprinkle the grated carrots over the hummus

3.Place slices of turkey over the sprinkled carrots.

4.Along the shorter edge of one end of the flatbread, line the olives in a row

5.Form the end with the olives, roll the flatbread

6.Slice across the long axis of the rolled bread into 4 pinwheels with a serrated knife (younger kids should seek their parents' assistance for safety).

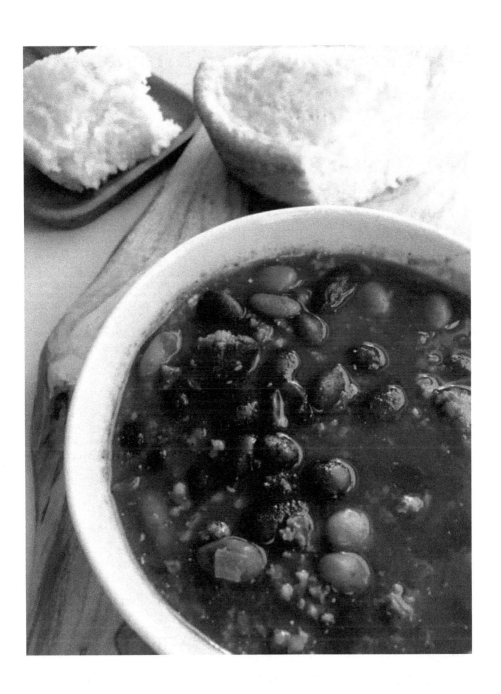

Mediterranean Chicken & Tomatoes

Total time: 35 minutes
Servings: 4

Ingredients:

1 pint Cherry tomatoes
1 package Chicken
1 pound Chicken breasts (skinless and boneless)
¼ cup Crumbled feta cheese
½ ounces Drained sliced black olives
1 tsp McCormick Oregano Leaves
1 tsp McCormick perfect pinch Italian seasoning
1 tsp Minced McCormick Garlic
2 tbsp Olive oil
½ tsp Salt

Directions:

1.The oven should be preheated to 450°F.

2.In a small bowl, mix all of the Spices and salt.

3.Place chicken, olives, tomatoes, and oil in large bowl.

4.Add the seasoning mixture;

5.Maneuver chicken in the large bowl to coat well.

6.Get a large but shallow baking pan and line with foil

7.Arrange chicken, tomatoes, and olives in one layer on the foil

8.Roast chicken for about 20 minutes or until chicken is cooked through or to taste

9.Sprinkle feta cheese on chicken

10.Serve hot

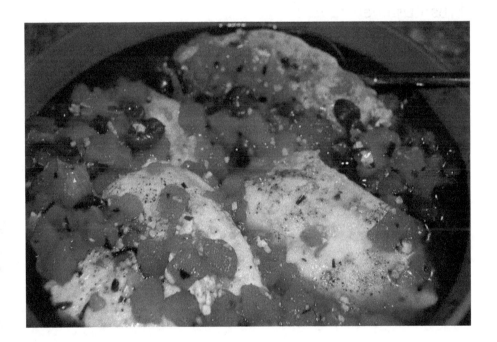

Mediterranean Chicken with Sun-Dried Tomatoes and Artichokes

Total time- 30 minutes
Servings: 4

Ingredients:

3 tbsp Drained capers
8 oz. Drained roasted artichoke hearts
¼ cup Flour (gluten-free flour can be used)
2 tbsp Freshly squeezed lemon juice
¼ tsp Ground black pepper
2 tbsp Olive oil
3 tbsp Olive oil
½ tsp Salt
6 oz Sun-dried tomatoes
1,5 pound Thin slices of chicken breast

Directions:

1.Chicken should be seasoned with salt and pepper.

2.Place chicken in a large plate, pour flour and properly coat chicken with it

3.Pour 2 tablespoons of olive oil in a large skillet over medium-high heat.

4.Add chicken and brown and wait for the mixture to turn golden about 4 minutes

5.Turn over the chicken and brown to the other side and heat for about 4 minutes on medium heat.

6.Take out the chicken unto the plate.

7.The add artichokes, sun-dried tomatoes, capers, and lemon juice to the same skillet.

8.Stir well until mixed adequately while heating over medium heat.

9.Tune down heat to low and add 2 or 3 tablespoons olive oil, further stir to mix well

10.Move aside the vegetables in the skillet and place back the chicken.

11.For about 5-10 minutes continuously cook the chicken and vegetables over low-medium heat, while covered.

12.Wait until chicken is properly cooked through, should not be pink on the inside

13.Serve while hot with the heated olive oil mixture over the chicken.

Mediterranean Turkey Chili

Total time:30 minutes
Servings: 4

Ingredients:

4 ounces Arugula leaves
2 cups Chicken stock
1 Chopped large Onion
Chopped Red chili pepper
4 ounces Crumbled Feta cheese
2 cans Diced tomatoes
2 cans Drained and rinsed white beans each)
2 cloves Finely chopped Garlic
1 pound Ground turkey
3 ounces Kalamata olives
3 tbsp Olive oil
3 ounces Thinly sliced Sun-dried tomatoes
1 tbsp Tomato paste

Directions:

1.Sieve the canned tomatoes, reserving just the juice.

2.Pour oil into a Dutch oven and heat over medium to high heat.

3.Add the ground turkey and sauté until it is brittle

4.Introduce onions, garlic, and chili pepper and sauté after about 2-3 minutes.

5.Add tomatoes paste to the mixture and stir while also adding stock sun-dried tomatoes and reserved tomato juice.

6.Increase the heat till the mixture starts to boil, then reduce heat to medium or low

7.Cover to allow the mixture to simmer for about 5 minutes.

8.After the 5 minutes, add the canned tomatoes, beans and olives and cook for an additional 5 minutes. Garnish with arugula, crumbled feta, and season chili.

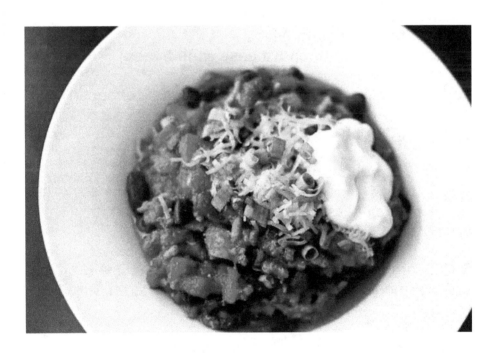

Mediterranean Chicken Macaroni and Cheese

Total time: 40 minutes
Servings: 4

Ingredients:

14 ½ ounces Quarters of chopped drained-artichoke hearts
1/3 cup Crumbled feta cheese
Fresh parsley
10 Chopped Kalamata olives
1 package Macaroni and cheese (Bob Evans)
2 cups Roasted chicken breast
½ cup Roasted and chopped red peppers (chopped)

Directions:

1.Start by preheating your oven to 375 °F

2.Get a small casserole dish and line with nonstick spray.

3.Mix combine the macaroni and cheese, chicken, artichoke hearts and peppers. Transfer the mixture into a dish

4.Sprinkle the mixture with feta and olives.

5.Place the dish into the oven to bake for about 25 to 30 minutes or microwave for 6 to 8 minutes, until it is cooked through.

6.Garnish macaroni and cheese with parsley

7.Serve hot.

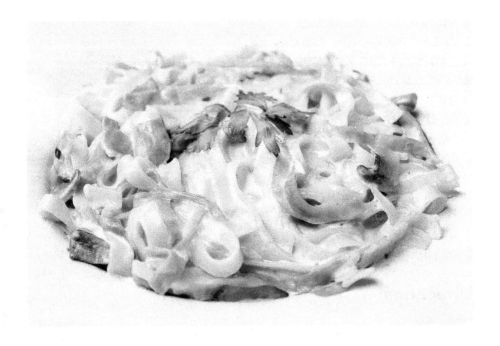

Rustic Vegetable and Brown Rice Bowl

Preparation Time: 15 minutes

Cooking Time: 10 minutes

Servings: 4

Ingredients:
Nonstick cooking spray
2 cups broccoli florets
1 cups cauliflower florets
1 (15-oz.) can chickpeas, drained and rinsed
1 cup carrots sliced
1 inch thick
2 to 3 tbsp. extra-virgin olive oil, divided
Salt and freshly ground black pepper
2 to 3 tbsp. sesame seeds, for garnish
2 cups cooked brown rice
3 to 4 tbsp. tahini
2 tbsp. honey
1 lemon, juiced
1 garlic clove, minced

Directions:

1.Preheat the oven to 400°F. Spray two baking sheets with cooking spray.

2.Cover the first baking sheet with the broccoli and cauliflower and the second with the chickpeas and carrots. Toss each sheet with half of the oil and season with salt and pepper before placing in oven.

3.Cook the carrots and chickpeas for 10 minutes, leaving the carrots still crisp, and the broccoli and cauliflower for 20 minutes, until tender. Stir each halfway through cooking.

4.In a small bowl, to make the dressing, mix the tahini, honey, lemon juice, and garlic. Season with salt and pepper and set aside.

5.Divide the rice into individual bowls, then layer with vegetables and drizzle dressing over the dish.

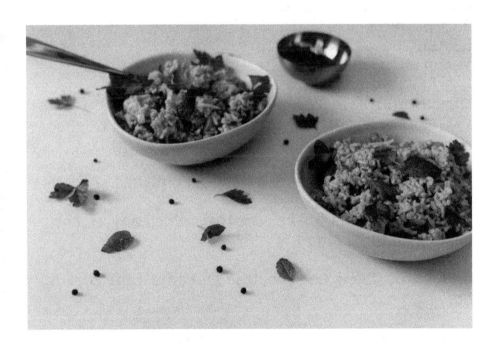

Roasted Brussels sprouts And Pecans

Preparation Time: 10 minutes

Cooking Time: 15 minute

Servings: 4

Ingredients:

1 ½ lb. fresh Brussels sprouts
4 tbsp. olive oil
4 cloves of garlic, minced
3 tbsp. water
Salt and pepper to taste
½ cup chopped pecans

Directions:

1.Place all ingredients in the Instant Pot.

2.Combine all ingredients until well combined.

3.Close the lid and make sure that the steam release vent is set to "Venting."

4.Press the "Slow Cook" button and adjust the cooking time to 3 hours.

5.Sprinkle with a dash of lemon juice if desired.

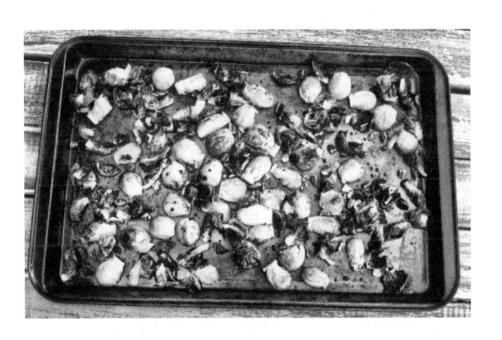

Eggs with Zucchini Noodles

Preparation Time: 10 minutes

Cooking Time: 11 minutes

Servings: 2

Ingredients:

2 tbsp. extra-virgin olive oil
3 zucchinis, cut with a spiralizer
4 eggs
Salt and black pepper to the taste
A pinch of red pepper flakes
Cooking spray
1 tbsp. basil, chopped

Directions:

1.In a bowl, combine the zucchini noodles with salt, pepper and the olive oil and toss well.

2.Grease a baking sheet with cooking spray and divide the zucchini noodles into 4 nests on it.

3.Crack an egg on top of each nest, sprinkle salt, pepper and the pepper flakes on top and bake at 350°F for 11 minutes.

4.Divide the mix between plates, sprinkle the basil on top and serve.

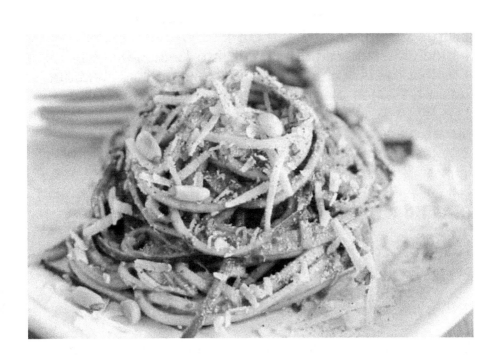

Roasted Root Veggies

Preparation Time: 20 minutes
Cooking Time: 1 hour 30 minute
Servings: 6

Ingredients:

2 tbsp. olive oil
1 head garlic, cloves separated and peeled
1 large turnip, peeled and cut into ½-inch pieces
1 medium sized red onion, cut into ½-inch pieces
1 ½ lbs. beets, trimmed but not peeled, scrubbed and cut into ½-inch pieces
1 ½ lbs. Yukon gold potatoes, unpeeled, cut into ½-inch pieces pieces
2 ½ lbs. butternut squash, peeled, seeded, cut into ½-inch

Directions:

1.Grease 2 rimmed and large baking sheets. Preheat oven to 425oF.

2.In a large bowl, mix all ingredients thoroughly.

3.Into the two baking sheets, evenly divide the root vegetables, spread in one layer.

4.Season generously with pepper and salt.

5.Pop into the oven and roast for 1 hour and 15 minute or until golden brown and tender.

6.Remove from oven and let it cool for at least 15 minutes before serving.

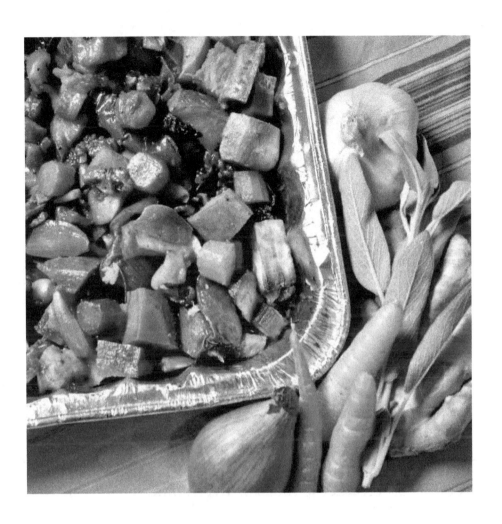

Roasted Vegetables and Zucchini Pasta

Preparation Time: 10 minutes

Cooking Time: 7 minute

Servings: 2

Ingredients:

¼ cup raw pine nuts
4 cups leftover vegetables
2 garlic cloves, minced
1 tbsp. extra virgin olive oil
4 medium zucchinis, cut into long strips resembling noodles

Directions:

1.Heat oil in a large skillet over medium heat and sauté the garlic for 2 minutes.

2.Add the leftover vegetables and place the zucchini noodles on top. Let it cook for five minutes. Garnish with pine nuts.

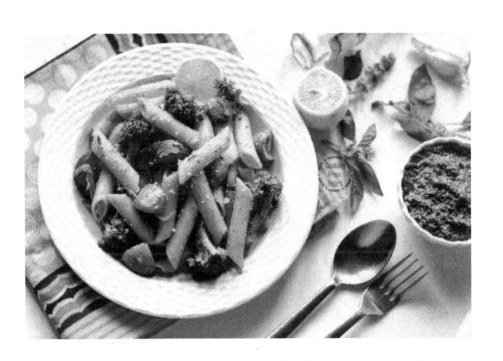

Sautéed Collard Greens

Preparation Time: 10 minutes

Cooking Time: 0 minute

Servings: 4

Ingredients:
1-lb. fresh collard greens, cut into
2-inch pieces 1 pinch red pepper flakes
3 cups chicken broth
1 tsp. pepper
1 tsp. salt
2 cloves garlic, minced
1 large onion, chopped
3 slices bacon
1 tbsp. olive oil

Directions:

1.Using a large skillet, heat oil on medium-high heat. Sauté bacon until crisp. Remove it from the pan and crumble it once cooled. Set it aside.

2.Using the same pan, sauté onion and cook until tender. Add garlic until fragrant. Add the collard greens and cook until they start to wilt.

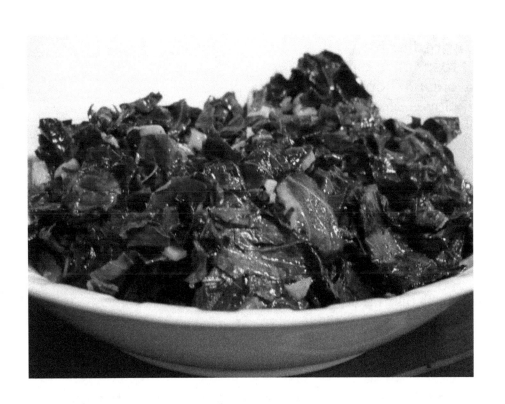

Savoy Cabbage with Coconut Cream Sauce

Preparation Time: 5 minutes

Cooking Time: 20 minute

Servings: 4

Ingredients:
3 tbsp. olive oil
1 onion, chopped
4 cloves of garlic, minced
1 head savoy cabbage, chopped finely
2 cups bone broth
1 cup coconut milk, freshly squeezed
1 bay leaf
Salt and pepper to taste
2 tbsp. chopped parsley

Directions:

1.Heat oil in a pot for 2 minutes.

2.Stir in the onions, bay leaf, and garlic until fragrant, around 3 minutes.

3.Add the rest of the ingredients, except for the parsley and mix well.

4.Cover pot, bring to a boil, and let it simmer for 5 minutes or until cabbage is tender to taste.

5.Stir in parsley and serve.

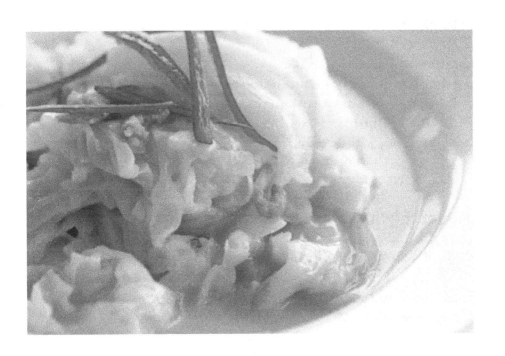

SlowCooked Buttery Mushrooms

Preparation Time: 10 minutes

Cooking Time: 10 minute

Servings: 2

Ingredients:

2 tbsp. butter
2 tbsp. olive oil
3 cloves of garlic, minced
16 oz. fresh brown mushrooms, sliced
7 oz. fresh shiitake mushrooms, sliced
A dash of thyme
Salt and pepper to taste

Directions:

1.Heat the butter and oil in a pot.

2.Sauté the garlic until fragrant, around 1 minute.

3.Stir in the rest of the ingredients and cook until soft, around 9 minutes.

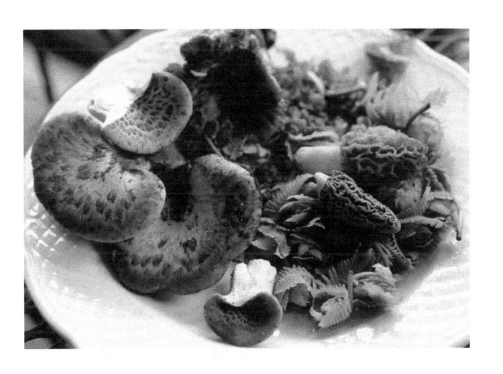

Steamed Squash Chowder

Preparation Time: 20 minutes

Cooking Time: 40 minute

Servings: 4

Ingredients:

3 cups chicken broth
2 tbsp. ghee
1 tsp. chili powder
½ tsp. cumin
1 ½ tsp. salt
2 tsp. cinnamon
3 tbsp. olive oil
2 carrots, chopped
1 small yellow onion, chopped
1 green apple, sliced and cored
1 large butternut squash, peeled, seeded, and chopped to ½-inch cubes

Directions:

1.In a large pot on medium high fire, melt ghee.

2.Once ghee is hot, sauté onions for 5 minutes or until soft and translucent.

3.Add olive oil, chili powder, cumin, salt, and cinnamon. Sauté for half a minute.

4.Add chopped squash and apples.

5.Sauté for 10 minutes while stirring once in a while.

6.Add broth, cover and cook on medium fire for twenty minutes or until apples and squash are tender.

7.With an immersion blender, puree chowder. Adjust consistency by adding more water.

8.Add more salt or pepper depending on desire.

9.Serve and enjoy.

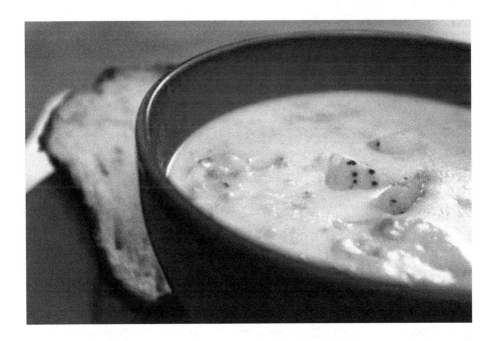

Steamed Zucchini-Paprika

Preparation Time: 15 minutes

Cooking Time: 30 minute

Servings: 2

Ingredients:

4 tbsp. olive oil
3 cloves of garlic, minced
1 onion, chopped
3 medium-sized zucchinis, sliced thinly
A dash of paprika
Salt and pepper to taste

Directions:

1.Place all ingredients in the Instant Pot.

2.Give a good stir to combine all ingredients.

3.Close the lid and make sure that the steam release valve is set to "Venting."

4.Press the "Slow Cook" button and adjust the cooking time to 4 hours.

5.Halfway through the cooking time, open the lid and give a good stir to brown the other side.

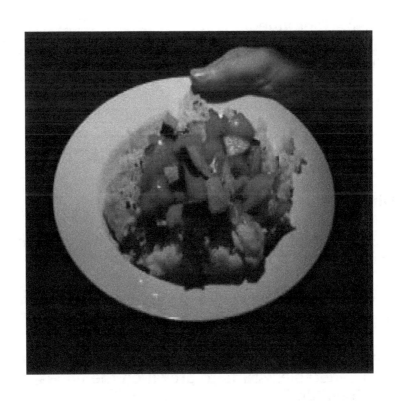

Stir Fried Brussels sprouts and Carrots

Preparation Time: 10 minutes

Cooking Time: 15 minute

Servings: 6

Ingredients:

1 tbsp. cider vinegar
1/3 cup water
1 lb. Brussels sprouts, halved lengthwise
1 lb. carrots cut diagonally into ½-inch thick lengths
3 tbsp. unsalted butter, divided
2 tbsp. chopped shallot
½ tsp. pepper
¾ tsp. salt

Directions:

1.On medium high fire, place a nonstick medium fry pan and heat 2 tbsp. butter.

2.Add shallots and cook until softened, around one to two minutes while occasionally stirring.

3.Add pepper salt, Brussels sprouts and carrots. Stir fry until vegetables starts to brown on the edges, around 3 to 4 minutes.

4.Add water, cook and cover.

5.After 5 to 8 minutes, or when veggies are already soft, add remaining butter.

6.If needed season with more pepper and salt to taste.

7.Turn off fire, transfer to a platter, serve and enjoy.

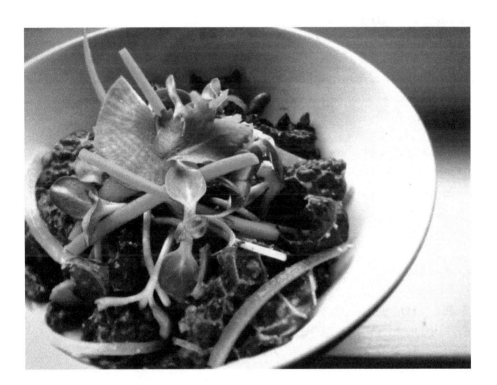

Stir Fried Eggplant Preparation

Preparations Time: 10 minutes
Cooking Time: 30 minute
Servings: 2

Ingredients:

1 tsp. cornstarch + 2 tbsp. water, mixed
1 tsp. brown sugar
2 tbsp. oyster sauce
1 tbsp. fish sauce
2 tbsp. soy sauce
½ cup fresh basil
2 tbsp. oil
¼ cup water
2 cups Chinese eggplant, spiral
1 red chili
6 cloves garlic, minced
½ purple onion, sliced thinly
1 3-oz package medium firm tofu, cut into slivers

Directions:

1.Prepare sauce by mixing cornstarch and water in a small bowl. In another bowl mix brown sugar, oyster sauce and fish sauce and set aside.

2.On medium high fire, place a large nonstick saucepan and heat 2 tbsp. oil. Sauté chili, garlic and onion for 4 minutes. Add tofu, stir fry for 4 minutes.

3.Add eggplant noodles and stir fry for 10 minutes. If pan dries up, add water in small amounts to moisten pan and cook noodles.

4.Pour in sauce and mix well. Once simmering, slowly add cornstarch mixer while continuing to mix vigorously. Once sauce thickens add fresh basil and cook for a minute.

5.Remove from fire, transfer to a serving plate and enjoy.

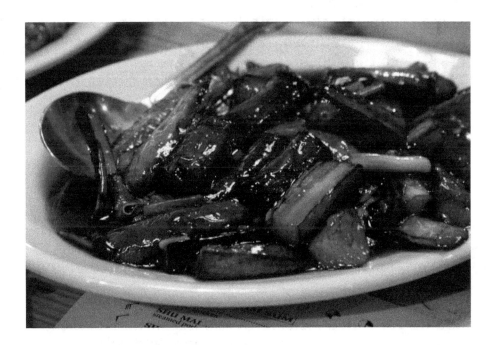

Summer Vegetables

Preparation Time: 20 minutes

Cooking Time: 1 hour 40 minutes minute
Servings: 6

Ingredients:

1 tsp. dried marjoram
1/3 cup Parmesan cheese
1 small eggplant, sliced into ¼-inch thick circles
1 small summer squash, peeled and sliced diagonally into ¼-inch thickness
3 large tomatoes, sliced into ¼-inch thick circles
½ cup dry white wine
½ tsp. freshly ground pepper, divided
½ tsp. salt, divided
5 cloves garlic, sliced thinly
2 cups leeks, sliced thinly
4 tbsp. extra virgin olive oil, divided

Directions:

1.On medium fire, place a large nonstick saucepan and heat 2 tbsp. oil.

2.Sauté garlic and leeks for 6 minutes or until garlic is starting to brown. Season with pepper and salt, ¼ tsp. each.

3.Pour in wine and cook for another minute. Transfer to a 2- quart baking dish.

4.In baking dish, layer in alternating pattern the eggplant, summer squash, and tomatoes. Do this until dish is covered with vegetables. If there are excess vegetables, store for future use.

5.Season with remaining pepper and salt. Drizzle with remaining olive oil and pop in a preheated 425oF oven.

6.Bake for 75 minutes. Remove from oven and top with marjoram and cheese.

7.Return to oven and bake for 15 minutes more or until veggies are soft and edges are browned.

8.Allow to cool for at least 5 minutes before serving.

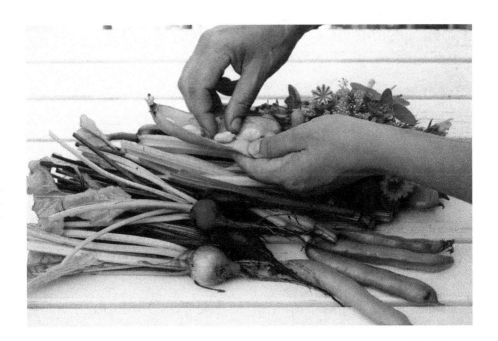

Stir Fried Bok Choy

Preparation Time: 5 minutes
Cooking Time: 13 minute
Servings: 4

Ingredients:

3 tbsp. coconut oil
4 cloves of garlic, minced
1 onion, chopped
2 heads bok choy, rinsed and chopped
2 tsp. coconut aminos
Salt and pepper to taste
2 tbsp. sesame oil
2 tbsp. sesame seeds, toasted

Directions:

1.Heat the oil in a pot for 2 minutes.

2.Sauté the garlic and onions until fragrant, around 3 minutes.

3.Stir in the bok choy, coconut aminos, salt and pepper.

4.Cover pan and cook for 5 minutes.

5.Stir and continue cooking for another 3 minutes.

6.Drizzle with sesame oil and sesame seeds on top before serving.

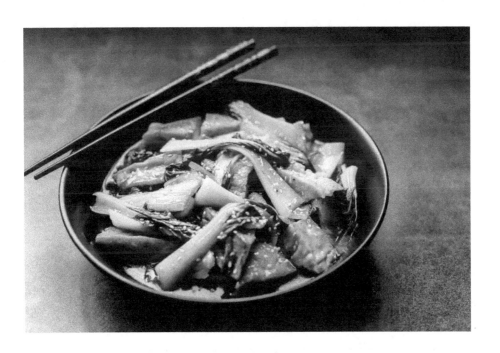

Summer Veggies in Instant Pot

Preparation Time: 10 minutes

Cooking Time: 7 minute

Servings: 6

Ingredients:

2 cups okra, sliced
1 cup grape tomatoes
1 cup mushroom, sliced 1 ½ cups onion, sliced
2 cups bell pepper, sliced 2 ½ cups zucchini, sliced
2 tbsp. basil, chopped
1 tbsp. thyme, chopped
½ cups balsamic vinegar
½ cups olive oil
Salt and pepper

Directions:

1.Place all ingredients in the Instant Pot.

2.Stir the contents and close the lid.

3.Close the lid and press the Manual button.

4.Adjust the cooking time to 7 minutes.

5.Do quick pressure release.

6.Once cooled, evenly divide into serving size, keep in your preferred container, and refrigerate until ready to eat.

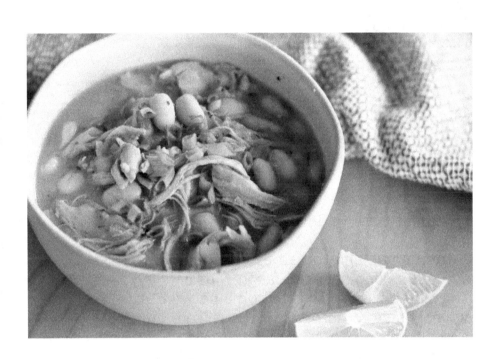

Sumptuous Tomato Soup

Preparation Time: 10 minutes

Cooking Time: 30 minute

Servings: 2

Ingredients:
Pepper and salt to taste
2 tbsp. tomato paste
1 ½ cups vegetable broth
1 tbsp. chopped parsley
1 tbsp. olive oil
5 garlic cloves
½ medium yellow onion
4 large ripe tomatoes

Directions:

1.Preheat oven to 350°F.

2.Chop onion and tomatoes into thin wedges. Place on a rimmed baking sheet. Season with parsley, pepper, salt, and olive oil. Toss to combine well. Hide the garlic cloves inside tomatoes to keep it from burning.

3.Pop in the oven and bake for 30 minutes.

4.On medium pot, bring vegetable stock to a simmer. Add tomato paste.

5.Pour baked tomato mixture into pot. Continue simmering for another 10 minutes.

6.With an immersion blender, puree soup.

7.Adjust salt and pepper to taste before serving.

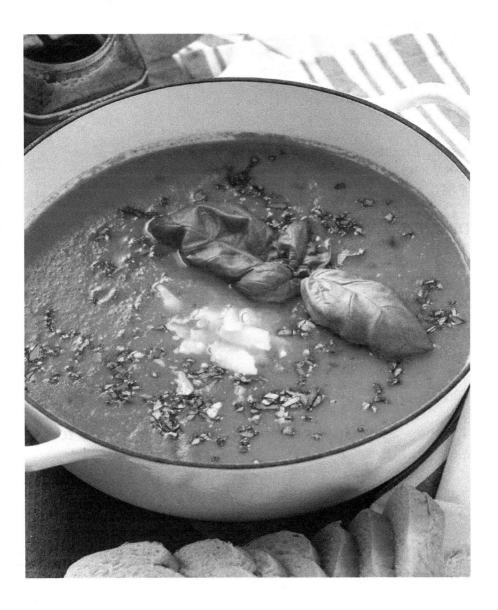

Superfast Cajun Asparagus

Preparation Time: 10 minutes

Cooking Time: 8 minute

Servings: 2

Ingredients:

1 tsp. Cajun seasoning
1-lb. asparagus
1 tsp. Olive oil

Directions:

1.Snap the asparagus and make sure that you use the tender part of the vegetable.

2.Place a large skillet on stovetop and heat on high for a minute.

3.Then grease skillet with cooking spray and spread asparagus in one layer.

4.Cover skillet and continue cooking on high for 5 to eight minutes.

5.Halfway through cooking time, stir skillet and then cover and continue to cook.

6.Once done cooking, transfer to plates, serve, and enjoy!

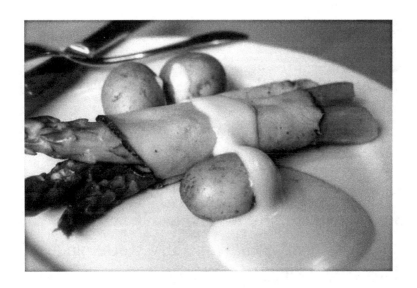

Sweet and Nutritious Pumpkin Soup

Preparation Time: 20 minutes

Cooking Time: 40 minute

Servings: 8

Ingredients:

1 tsp. chopped fresh parsley
½ cup half and half
½ tsp. chopped fresh thyme
1 tsp. salt
4 cups pumpkin puree
6 cups vegetable stock, divided
1 clove garlic, minced
1 1-inch piece gingerroot, peeled and minced
   1 cup chopped onion

Directions:

1.On medium high fire, place a heavy bottomed pot and for 5 minutes heat ½ cup vegetable stock, ginger, garlic and onions or until veggies are tender.

2.Add remaining stock and cook for 30 minutes.

3.Season with thyme and salt.

4.With an immersion blender, puree soup until smooth.

5.Turn off fire and mix in half and half.

7.Transfer pumpkin soup into 8 bowls, garnish with parsley, serve and enjoy.

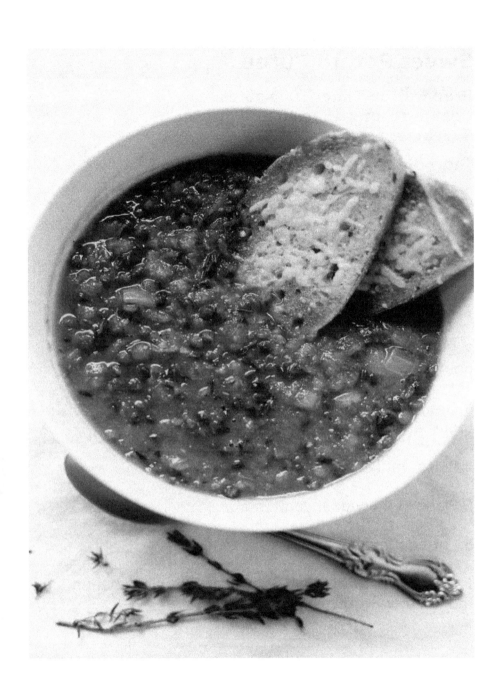

Sweet Potato Puree

Preparation Time: 10 minutes
Cooking Time: 15 minute
Servings: 6

Ingredients:

2lb. sweet potatoes, peeled
1 ½ cups water
5 Medjool dates, pitted and chopped

Directions:

1.Place all ingredients in a pot.

2.Close the lid and allow to boil for 15 minutes until the potatoes are soft.

3.Drain the potatoes and place in a food processor together with the dates.

4.Pulse until smooth.

5.Place in individual containers.

6.Put a label and store in the fridge.

7.Allow to thaw at room temperature before heating in the microwave oven.

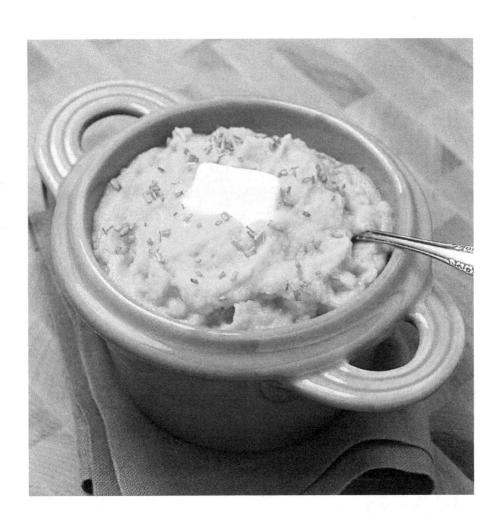

Sweet Potato Soup

Preparation Time: 10 minutes
Cooking Time: 30 minute
Servings: 4

Ingredients:

2tbsp Pepper and salt to taste
2thyme leaves Juice of half a lemon
1tsp. ground cumin
2cups mashed sweet potato
4 cups chicken stock
4 bell pepper, diced
1 onion, diced
1 tbsp. coconut oil

Directions:

1.On medium low fire, place a heavy bottomed pot and heat coconut oil.

2.Sauté peppers and onions for 5 minutes or until slightly soft.

3.Meanwhile, in a blender puree mashed sweet potatoes with 2 cups chicken stock. Pour into pot.

4.Add cumin and remaining chicken stock. Cover and bring to a boil.

5.Lower fire to a simmer and cook for 20 minutes or until peppers are tender.

6.Season with pepper, salt, thyme and lemon juice. Serve while hot.

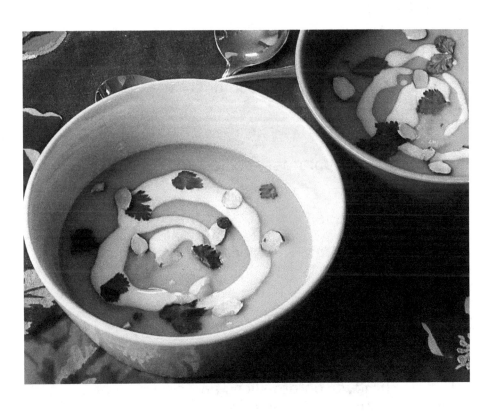

Sweet Potatoes Oven Fried

Preparation Time: 10 minutes

Cooking Time: 30 minute

Servings: 7

Ingredients:

1 small garlic clove, minced
1 tsp. grated orange rind
1 tbsp. fresh parsley, chopped finely
¼ tsp. pepper
¼ tsp. salt
1 tbsp. olive oil
4 medium sweet potatoes, peeled and sliced to ¼-inch thickness

Directions:

1.In a large bowl mix well pepper, salt, olive oil and sweet potatoes.

2.In a greased baking sheet, in a single layer arrange sweet potatoes.

3.Pop in a preheated 400oF oven and bake for 15 minutes, turnover potato slices and return to oven. Bake for another 15 minutes or until tender.

4.Meanwhile, mix well in a small bowl garlic, orange rind and parsley, sprinkle over cooked potato slices and serve.

5.You can store baked sweet potatoes in a lidded container and just microwave whenever you want to eat it. Do consume within 3 days.

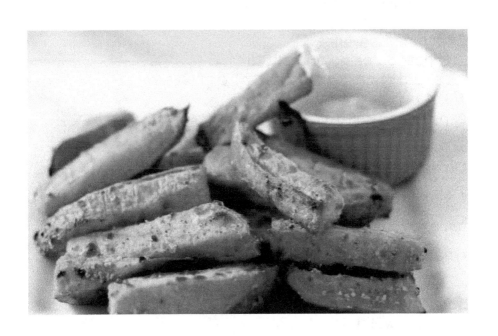

Tasty Avocado Sauce over Zoodles

Preparation Time: 10 minutes

Cooking Time: 10 minute

Servings: 2

Ingredients:

1 zucchini peeled and spiralized into noodles
4 tbsp. pine nuts
2 tbsp. lemon juice
1 avocado peeled and pitted
12 sliced cherry tomatoes 1/3 cup water
1 1/4 cup basil
Pepper and salt to taste

Directions:

1.Make the sauce in a blender by adding pine nuts, lemon juice, avocado, water, and basil. Pulse until smooth and creamy. Season with pepper and salt to taste. Mix well.

2.Place zoodles in salad bowl. Pour over avocado sauce and toss well to coat.

3.Add cherry tomatoes, serve, and enjoy.

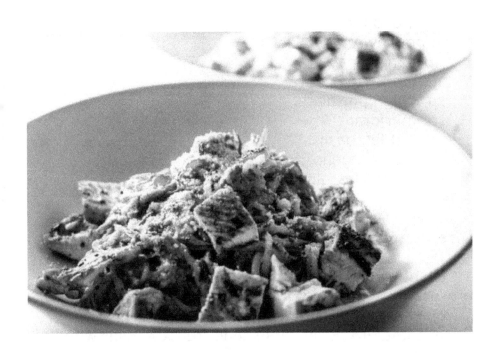

Tomato Basil Cauliflower Rice

Preparation Time: 5 minutes

Cooking Time: 10 minute

Servings: 4

Ingredients:

Salt and pepper to taste
Dried parsley for garnish
¼ cup tomato paste
½ tsp. garlic, minced
½ tsp. onion powder
½ tsp. marjoram
1 ½ tsp. dried basil
1 tsp. dried oregano
1 large head of cauliflower
1 tsp. oil

Directions:

1.Cut the cauliflower into florets and place in the food processor.

2.Pulse until it has a coarse consistency similar with rice. Set aside.

3.In a skillet, heat the oil and sauté the garlic and onion for three minutes. Add the rest of the ingredients. Cook for 8 minutes.

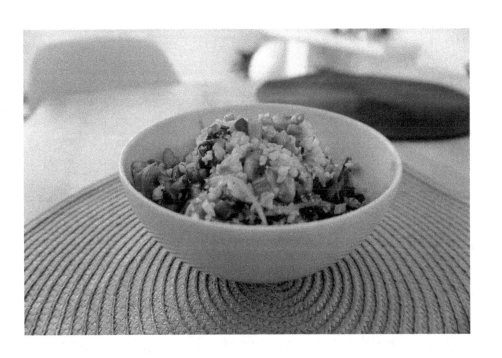

Vegan Sesame Tofu and Eggplants

Preparation Time: 10 minutes

Cooking Time: 20 minute

Servings: 4

Ingredients:

5tbsp. olive oil
1lb. firm tofu, sliced
3tbsp. rice vinegar
2tsp. Swerve sweetener
2 whole eggplants, sliced
¼ cup soy sauce
Salt and pepper to taste
4 tbsp. toasted sesame oil
¼ cup sesame seeds
1 cup fresh cilantro, chopped

Directions:

1.Heat the oil in a pan for 2 minutes.

2.Pan fry the tofu for 3 minutes on each side.

3.Stir in the rice vinegar, sweetener, eggplants, and soy sauce. Season with salt and pepper to taste.

4.Cover and cook for 5 minutes on medium fire. Stir and continue cooking for another 5 minutes.

5.Toss in the sesame oil, sesame seeds, and cilantro.

6.Serve and enjoy.

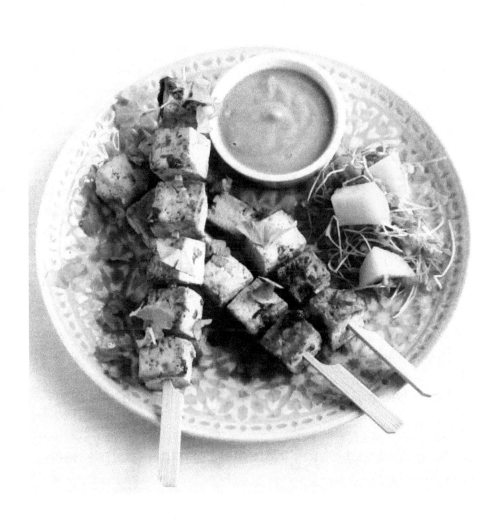

77

Vegetarian Coconut Curry

Preparation Time: 10 minutes

Cooking Time: 30 minute

Servings: 4

Ingredients:

4tbsp. coconut oil
1medium onion, chopped
1tsp. minced garlic
1tsp. minced ginger
1cup broccoli florets
2cups fresh spinach leaves
2 tsp. fish sauce
1 tbsp. garam masala
½ cup coconut milk
Salt and pepper to taste

Directions:

1.Heat oil in a pot.

2.Sauté the onion and garlic until fragrant, around 3 minutes.

3.Stir in the rest of the ingredients, except for spinach leaves.

4.Season with salt and pepper to taste.

5.Cover and cook on medium fire for 5 minutes.

6.Stir and add spinach leaves. Cover and cook for another 2 minutes.

7.Turn off fire and let it sit for two more minutes before serving.

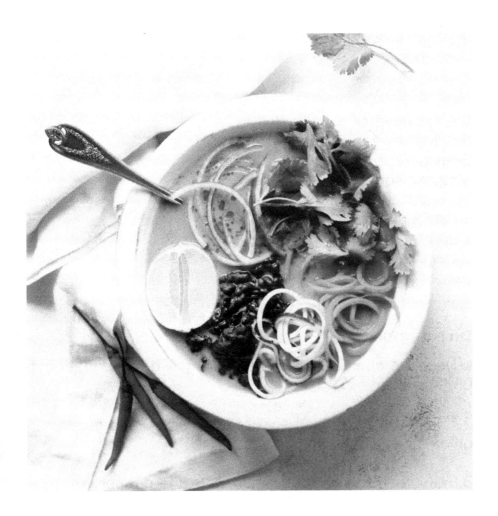

Veggie Lo Mein

Preparation Time: 10 minutes
Cooking Time: 4 minute
Servings: 6

Ingredients:

2 tbsp. olive oil
5 cloves of garlic, minced
2- inch knob of ginger, grated
8 oz. mushrooms, sliced
½ lb. zucchini, spiralized
1 carrot, julienned
1 spring green onions, chopped
3 tbsp. coconut aminos
Salt and pepper to taste
1 tbsp. sesame oil

Directions:

1.Heat the oil in a skillet and sauté the garlic and ginger until fragrant.

2.Stir in the mushrooms, zucchini, carrot, and green onions.

3.Season with coconut aminos, salt and pepper.

4.Close the lid and allow to simmer for 5 minutes.

5.Drizzle with sesame oil last.

6.Place in individual containers.

7.Put a label and store in the fridge.

8.Allow to thaw at room temperature before heating in the microwave oven

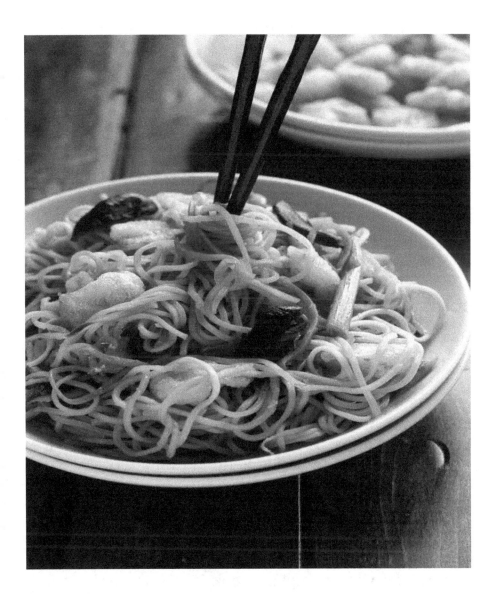

Veggie Jamaican Stew Preparation

Preparation Time: 15 minutes
Cooking Time: 30 minute
Servings: 4

Ingredients:

1 tbsp. cilantro, chopped
1 tsp. salt
1 tsp. pepper
1 tbsp. lime juice
2 cups collard greens, sliced
3 cups carrots, cut into bite-sized chunks
½ yellow plantain, cut into bite-sized pieces
1cup okra, cut into ½" pieces
2cups potatoes, cut into bite-sized cubes
2cups taro, cut into bite sized cubes
2cups pumpkin, cut into bite sized cubes
2 cups water
2 cups coconut milk

Directions:

1.On medium fire, place a stockpot and heat oil. Sauté onions for 4 minutes or until translucent and soft. Add thyme, all spice and garlic. Sauté for a minute.

2.Pour in water and coconut milk and bring to a simmer. Add bay leaves and green onions.

3.Once simmering, slow fire to keep broth at a simmer and add taro and pumpkin. Cook for 5 minutes.

4.Add potatoes and cook for three minutes.

5.Add carrots, plantain and okra. Mix and cook for five minutes.

6.Then remove and fish for thyme sprigs, bay leaves and green onions and discard.

7.Add collard greens and cook for four minutes or until bright green and darker in color.

8.Turn off fire, add pepper, salt and lime juice to taste. Once it tastes good, mix well, transfer to a serving bowl, serve and enjoy.

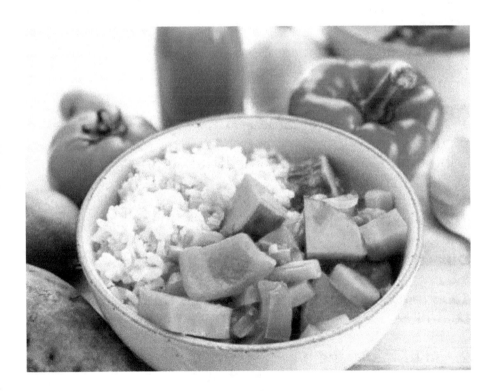

Vegetable Soup Moroccan Style

Preparation Time: 10 minutes

Cooking Time: 10 minute

Servings: 6

Ingredients:

½ tsp. pepper
1 tsp. salt
2 oz whole wheat orzo
1 large zucchini, peeled and cut into ¼-insh cubes
8 sprigs fresh cilantro, plus more leaves for garnish
12 sprigs flat leaf parsley, plus more for garnish
A pinch of saffron threads
2stalks celery leaves included, sliced thinly
2carrots, diced
2small turnips, peeled and diced
1 14-oz can diced tomatoes
6 cups water
1 lb. lamb stew meat, trimmed and cut into ½-inch
cubes 2 tsp. ground turmeric
1 medium onion, diced finely
2 tbsp. extra virgin olive oil

Directions:

1.On medium high fire, place a large Dutch oven and heat oil.

2.Add turmeric and onion, stir fry for two minutes.

3.Add meat and sauté for 5 minutes.

4.Add saffron, celery, carrots, turnips, tomatoes and juice, and water.

5.With a kitchen string, tie cilantro and parsley sprigs together and into pot.

6.Cover and bring to a boil. Once boiling reduce fire to a simmer and continue to cook for 45 to 50 minutes or until meat is tender.

7.Once meat is tender, stir in zucchini. Cover and cook for 8 minutes.

8.Add orzo; cook for 10 minutes or until soft.

9.Remove and discard cilantro and parsley sprigs.

10.Season with pepper and salt.

11.Transfer to a serving bowl and garnish with cilantro and parsley leaves before serving.

Veggie Ramen Miso Soup

Preparation Time: 5 minutes

Cooking Time: 20 minute

Servings: 1

Ingredients:
2tsp. thinly sliced green onion
A pinch of salt
½ tsp. shoyu
2 tbsp. mellow white miso
1 cup zucchini, cut into angel hair spirals
½ cup thinly sliced cremini mushrooms
½ medium carrot, cut into angel hair spirals
1/2 cup baby spinach leaves – optional
2 ¼ cups water
½ box of medium firm tofu, cut into ¼-inch cubes
1 hardboiled egg

Directions:

1.In a small bowl, mix ¼ cup of water and miso. Set aside.

2.In a small saucepan on medium high fire, bring to a boil 2 cups water, mushrooms, tofu and carrots. Add salt, shoyu and miso mixture.

3.Allow to boil for 5 minutes. Remove from fire and add green onion, zucchini and baby spinach leaves if using.

4.Let soup stand for 5 minutes before transferring to individual bowls. Garnish with ½ of hardboiled egg per bowl, serve and enjoy.

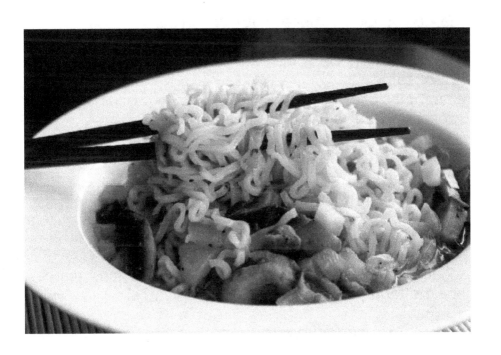

Yummy Cauliflower Fritters

Preparation Time: 10 minutes

Cooking Time: 15 minute

Servings: 6

Ingredients:

1 large cauliflower head, cut into florets
2 eggs, beaten
½ tsp. turmeric
½ tsp. salt
¼ tsp. black pepper
6 tbsp. coconut oil

Directions:

1.Place the cauliflower florets in a pot with water.

2.Bring to a boil and drain once cooked.

3.Place the cauliflower, eggs, turmeric, salt, and pepper into the food processor.

4.Pulse until the mixture becomes coarse.

5.Transfer into a bowl. Using your hands, form six small flattened balls and place in the fridge for at least 1 hour until the mixture hardens.

6.Heat the oil in a skillet and fry the cauliflower patties for 3 minutes on each side

7.Place in individual containers.

8.Put a label and store in the fridge.

9.Allow to thaw at room temperature before heating in the microwave oven.

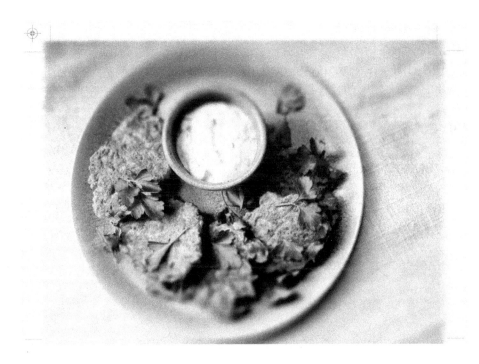

Zucchini Garlic Fries

Preparation Time: 15 minutes
Cooking Time: 20 minute
Servings: 6

Ingredients:

¼ tsp. garlic powder
½ cup almond flour
2large egg whites, beaten
2medium zucchinis, sliced into fry sticks
Salt and pepper to taste

Directions:

1.Preheat oven to 400°F.

2.Mix all ingredients in a bowl until the zucchini fries are well coated.

3.Place fries on cookie sheet and spread evenly.

4.Put in oven and cook for 20 minutes.

5.Halfway through cooking time, stir fries.

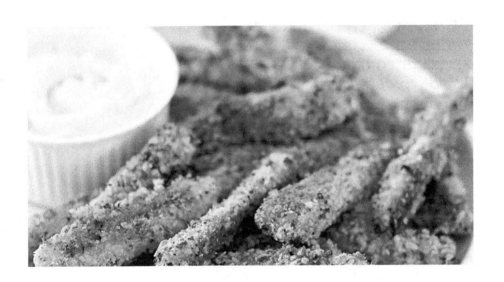

Zucchini Pasta with Mango-Kiwi Sauce

Preparation Time: 5 minutes

Cooking Time: 20 minute

Servings: 2

Ingredients:

1 tsp. dried herbs – optional
½ Cup Raw Kale leaves, shredded
2small dried figs
2medjool dates
4medium kiwis
2big mangos, seed discarded
2 cup zucchini, spiralized
¼ cup roasted cashew

Directions:

1.On a salad bowl, place kale then topped with zucchini noodles and sprinkle with dried herbs. Set aside.

2.In a food processor, grind to a powder the cashews. Add figs, dates, kiwis and mangoes then puree to a smooth consistency.

3.Pour over zucchini pasta, serve and enjoy.

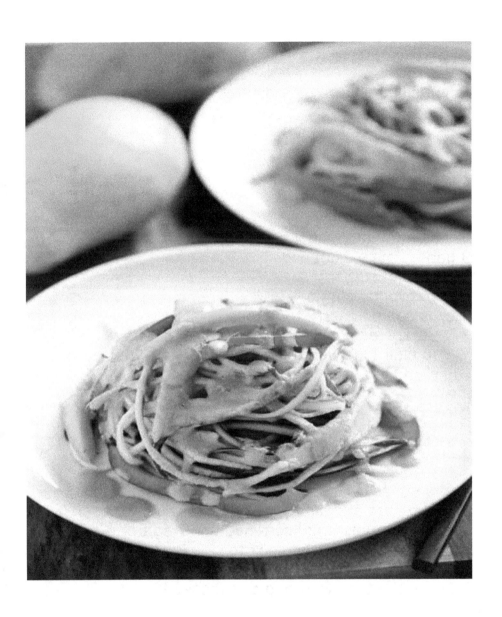

Mediterranean Baked Chickpeas

Preparation Time: 15 minutes

Coooking Time: 15 minute

Servings: 6

Ingredients:

1 tbsp. extra-virgin olive oil
½ medium onion, chopped
3 garlic cloves, chopped
2 tsp. smoked paprika
¼ tsp. ground cumin
4 cups halved cherry tomatoes
2 (15-oz.) cans chickpeas, drained and rinsed
½ cup plain, unsweetened, full-fat Greek yogurt, for 1 cup crumbled feta, for serving

Directions:

1.Preheat the oven to 425°F.

2.In an oven-safe sauté pan or skillet, heat the oil over medium heat and sauté the onion and garlic. Cook for about 5 minutes, until softened and fragrant. Stir in the paprika and cumin and cook for 2 minutes.

3.Stir in the tomatoes and chickpeas.

4.Bring to a simmer for 5 to 10 minutes before placing in the oven.

5.Roast in oven for 25 to 30 minutes, until bubbling and thickened. To serve, top with Greek yogurt and feta.

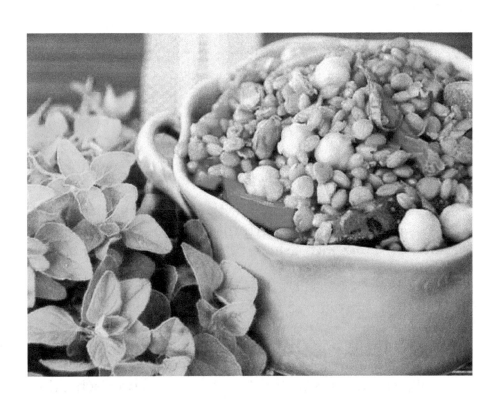

Falafel Bites

Preparation Time: 10 minutes
Cooking Time: 15 minute
Servings: 4

Ingredients:

1 2/3 cups falafel mix
1¼ cups water
Extra-virgin olive oil spray
1 tbsp. Pickled Onions (optional)
1 tbsp. Pickled Turnips (optional)
2 tbsp. Tzatziki Sauce (optional)

Directions:

1.In a large bowl, carefully stir the falafel mix into the water. Mix well. Let stand 15 minutes to absorb the water. Form mix into 1-inch balls and arrange on a baking sheet.

2.Preheat the broiler to high.

3.Take the balls and flatten slightly with your thumb (so they won't roll around on the baking sheet). Spray with olive oil, and then broil for 2 to 3 minutes on each side, until crispy and brown.

4.To fry the falafel, fill a pot with ½ inch of cooking oil and heat over medium-high heat to 375°F. Fry the balls for about3 minutes, until brown and crisp. Drain on paper towels and serve with pickled onions, pickled turnips, and tzatziki sauce (if using).

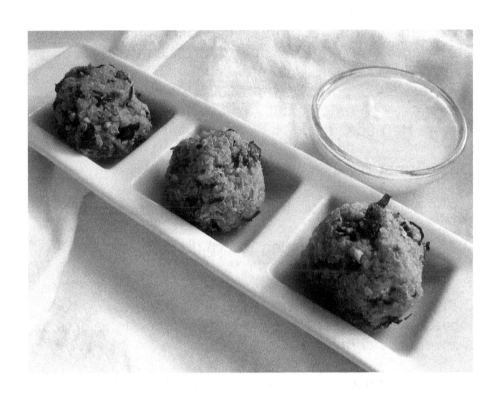

Quick Vegetable Kebabs

Preparation Time: 15 minutes
Cooking Time: 20 minute
Servings: 6

Ingredients:

4medium red onions, peeled and sliced into 6 wedges
4medium zucchini, cut into 1-inch-thick slices
4bell peppers, cut into 2-inch squares
2yellow bell peppers, cut into 2-inch squares
2orange bell peppers, cut into 2-inch squares
2 beefsteak tomatoes, cut into quarters
3 tbsp. Herbed Oil

Directions:

1.Preheat the oven or grill to medium-high or 350°F.

2.Thread 1 piece red onion, zucchini, different colored bell peppers, and tomatoes onto a skewer.

3.Repeat until the skewer is full of vegetables, up to 2 inches away from the skewer end, and continue until all skewers are complete.

4.Put the skewers on a baking sheet and cook in the oven for 10 minutes or grill for 5 minutes on each side. The vegetables will be done with they reach your desired crunch or softness.

5.Remove the skewers from heat and drizzle with Herbed Oil.

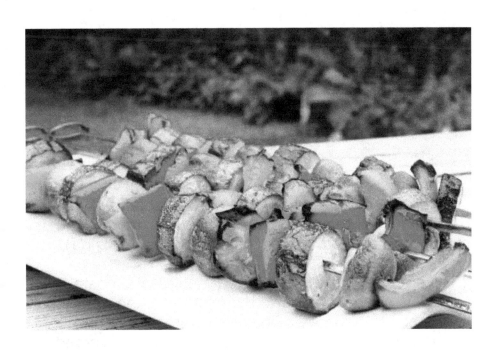

Tortellini in Red Pepper Sauce

Preparation Time: 15 minutes

Cooking Time: 10 minute

Servings: 4

Ingredients:

1 container fresh cheese tortellini (usually green
and white pasta)
1 roasted red peppers, drained
1 tsp. garlic powder
¼ cup tahini
1 tbsp. red pepper oil (optional)

Directions:

1.In a blender, combine the red peppers with the garlic powder and process until smooth. Once blended, add the tahini until the sauce is thickened. If the sauce gets too thick, add up to 1 tbsp. red pepper oil (if using).

2.Once tortellini are cooked, drain and leave pasta in colander. Add the sauce to the bottom of the empty pot and heat for 2 minutes. Then, add the tortellini back into the pot and cook for 2 more minutes. Serve and enjoy!

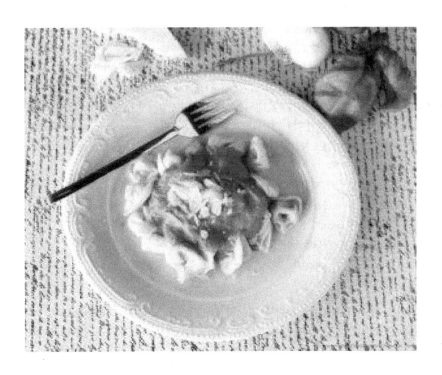

Freekeh, Chickpea, and Herb Salad

Preparation Time: 15 minutes

Cooking Time: 10 minute

Servings: 6

Ingredients:

1 (15-oz.) can chickpeas, rinsed and drained
1 cup cooked freekeh
1 cup thinly sliced celery
1 bunch scallions, both white and green parts, finely chopped
½ cup chopped fresh flat-leaf parsley
¼ cup chopped fresh mint
2tbsp. chopped celery leaves
½ tsp. kosher salt
1/3 cup extra-virgin olive oil
¼ cup freshly squeezed lemon juice
¼ tsp. cumin seeds
1 tsp. garlic powder

Directions:

1.In a large bowl, combine the chickpeas, freekeh, celery, scallions, parsley, mint, celery leaves, and salt and toss lightly.

2.In a small bowl, whisk together the olive oil, lemon juice, cumin seeds, and garlic powder. Once combined, add to freekeh salad.

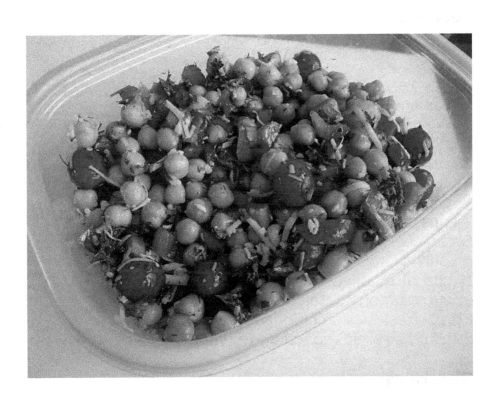

Kate's Warm Mediterranean Farro Bowl

Preparation Time: 15 minutes

Cooking Time: 10 minute

Servings: 4

Ingredients:

1/3 cup extra-virgin olive oil
½ cup chopped red bell pepper
1/3 cup chopped red onions
2 garlic cloves, minced
1 cup zucchini, cut in ½-inch slices
½ cup canned chickpeas, drained and rinsed
½ cup coarsely chopped artichokes
3 cups cooked farro
Salt
Freshly ground black pepper
¼ cup sliced olives, for serving
½ cup crumbled feta cheese, for serving
2tbsp. fresh basil, chiffonade, for serving
3 tbsp. balsamic reduction, for serving

Directions:

1.In a large sauté pan or skillet, heat the oil over medium heat and sauté the pepper, onions, and garlic for about 5 minutes, until tender.

2.Add the zucchini, chickpeas, and artichokes, then stir and continue to sauté vegetables, approximately 5 more minutes, until just soft.

3.Stir in the cooked farro, tossing to combine and cooking enough to heat through. Season with salt and peepper and remove from the heat.

4.Transfer the contents of the pan into the serving vessels or bowls.

5.Top with olives, feta, and basil (if using). Drizzle with balsamic reduction (if using) to finish.

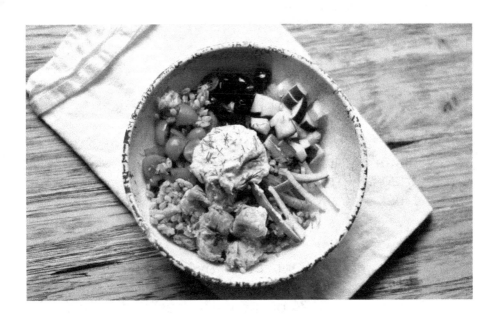

Creamy Chickpea Sauce with Whole-Wheat Fusilli

Preparation Time: 15 minutes

Cooking Time: 20 minute

Servings: 4

Ingredients:

¼ cup extra-virgin olive oil
½ large shallot, chopped
5garlic cloves, thinly sliced
1can chickpeas, drained and rinsed, reserving
½ cup canning liquid
Pinch red pepper flakes
1 cup whole-grain fusilli pasta
¼ tsp. salt
1/8 tsp. freshly ground black pepper
¼ cup shaved fresh Parmesan cheese
¼ cup chopped fresh basil
2 tsp. dried parsley
1 tsp. dried oregano Red pepper flakes

Directions:

1.In a medium pan, heat the oil over medium heat, and sauté the shallot and garlic for 3 to 5 minutes, until the garlic is golden. Add ¾ of the chickpeas plus 2 tbsp. of liquid from the can, and bring to a simmer.

2.Remove from the heat, transfer into a standard blender, and blend until smooth. At this point, add the remaining chickpeas. Add more reserved chickpea liquid if it becomes thick.

3.Bring a large pot of salted water to a boil and cook pasta until al dente, about 8 minutes. Reserve ½ cup of the pasta water, drain the pasta, and return it to the pot.

4.Add the chickpea sauce to the hot pasta and add up to ¼ cup of the pasta water. You may need to add more pasta water to reach your desired consistency.

5.Place the pasta pot over medium heat and mix occasionally until the sauce thickens. Season with salt and pepper.

6.Serve, garnished with Parmesan, basil, parsley, oregano, and red pepper flakes.

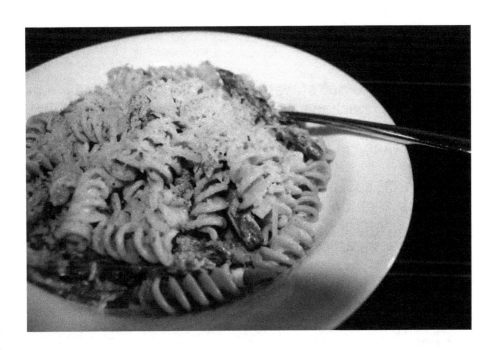

Linguine and Brussels sprouts

Preparation Time: 10 minutes

Cooking Time: 25 minute

Servings: 4

Ingredients:
8 oz. whole-wheat linguine
1/3 cup, plus
2tbsp. extra-virgin olive oil, divided
1 medium sweet onion, diced
2 to 3 garlic cloves, smashed
8 oz. Brussels sprouts, chopped
½ cup chicken stock, as needed
1/3 cup dry white wine
½ cup shredded Parmesan cheese
1 lemon, cut in quarters

Directions:

1.Bring a large pot of water to a boil and cook the pasta according to package directions. Drain, reserving 1 cup of the pasta water. Mix the cooked pasta with 2 tbsp. of olive oil, then set aside.

2.In a large sauté pan or skillet, heat the remaining 1/3 cup of olive oil on medium heat. Add the onion to the pan and cook for about 5 minutes, until softened. Add the smashed garlic cloves and cook for 1 minute, until fragrant.

3.Add the Brussels sprouts and cook covered for 15 minutes. Add chicken stock as needed to prevent burning.

4.Once Brussels sprouts have wilted and are fork-tender, add white wine and cook down for about 7 minutes, until reduced.

5.Add the pasta to the skillet and add the pasta water as needed.

6.Serve with the Parmesan cheese and lemon for squeezing over the dish right before eating.

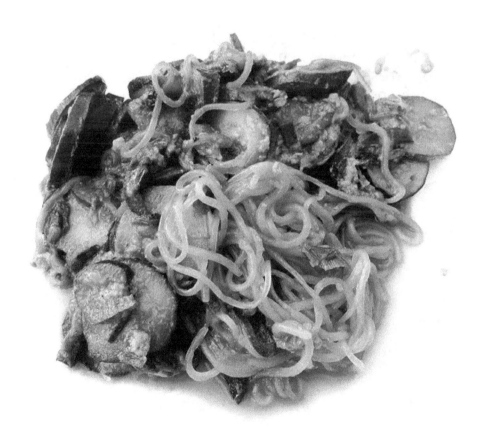

Peppers and Lentils Salad

Preparation Time: 10 minutes
Cooking Time: 0 minutes
Servings: 4

Ingredients:

14 oz. canned lentils, drained and rinsed
2 spring onions, chopped
1 red bell pepper, chopped
1 green bell pepper, chopped
1 tbsp. fresh lime juice
1/3 cup coriander, chopped
2tsp. balsamic vinegar

Directions:

1.In a salad bowl, combine the lentils with the onions, bell peppers and the rest of the ingredients, toss and serve.

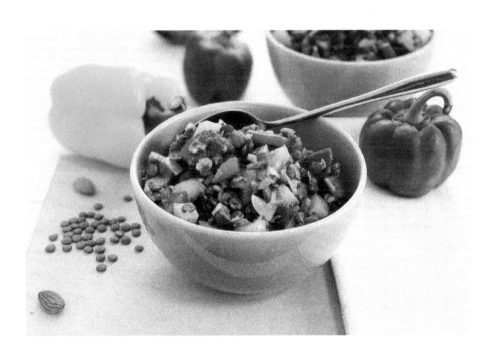

Cashews and Red Cabbage Salad

Preparation Time: 10 minutes
Cooking Time: 0 minutes
Servings: 4

Ingredients:

1 lb. red cabbage, shredded
2 tbsp. coriander, chopped
½ cup cashews, halved
2 tbsp. olive oil
1 tomato, cubed
A pinch of salt and black pepper
1 tbsp. white vinegar

Directions:

1.In a salad bowl, combine the cabbage with the coriander and the rest of the ingredients, toss and serve cold.

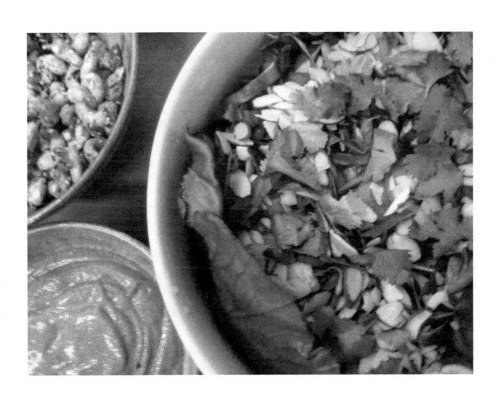

CPSIA information can be obtained
at www.ICGtesting.com
Printed in the USA
BVHW092324270421
605944BV00004B/637